This Health Hazard Evaluation (HHE) report and any recommendations made herein are for the specific facility evaluated and may not be universally applicable. Any recommendations made are not to be considered as final statements of NIOSH policy or of any agency or individual involved. Additional HHE reports are available at http://www.cdc.gov/niosh/hhe/

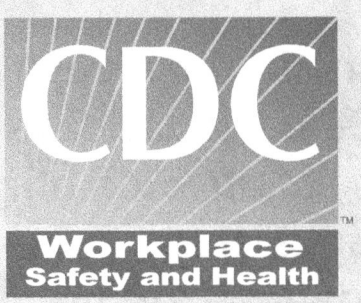

I0426382

# Evaluation of Methicillin-resistant *Staphylococcus aureus* (MRSA) Cases among Employees at a Workholding Manufacturing Facility

*John Gibbins, DVM, MPH*
*Todd Niemeier, MS, CIH*

Health Hazard Evaluation Report
HETA 2009-0098-3103
Positrol Inc.
Cincinnati, Ohio
March 2010

Department of Health and Human Services
Centers for Disease Control and Prevention

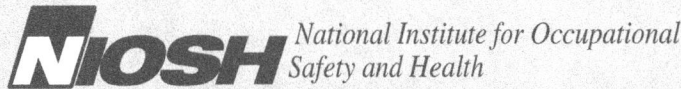 *National Institute for Occupational Safety and Health*

The employer shall post a copy of this report for a period of 30 calendar days at or near the workplace(s) of affected employees. The employer shall take steps to insure that the posted determinations are not altered, defaced, or covered by other material during such period. [37 FR 23640, November 7, 1972, as amended at 45 FR 2653, January 14, 1980].

# CONTENTS

# ABBREVIATIONS

| | |
|---|---|
| °C | Degrees celsius |
| CFU | Colony forming unit |
| cm | Centimeter |
| cm$^2$ | Square centimeter |
| EPA | Environmental Protection Agency |
| HEPA | High efficiency particulate air |
| HHE | Health hazard evaluation |
| HP | Hypersensitivity pneumonitis |
| HSE | Health and Safety Executive |
| IARC | International Agency for Research on Cancer |
| MWF | Metalworking fluid |
| mg/m$^3$ | Milligrams per cubic meter |
| mL | Milliliter |
| MRSA | Methicillin-resistant *Staphylococcus aureus* |
| NAICS | North American Industry Classification System |
| NIOSH | National Institute for Occupational Safety and Health |
| OSHA | Occupational Safety and Health Administration |
| PAH | Polycyclic aromatic hydrocarbon |
| PEL | Permissible exposure limit |
| PPE | Personal protective equipment |
| REL | Recommended exposure limit |
| STEL | Short-term exposure limit |
| TWA | Time-weighted average |

In February 2009, the National Institute for Occupational Safety and Health (NIOSH) received a management request for a health hazard evaluation at Positrol Inc. in Cincinnati, Ohio. The company submitted the request because several employees had reported methicillin-resistant *Staphylococcus aureus* (MRSA) skin infections, and management wanted to determine if these infections were related to workplace exposures.

## What NIOSH Did

- We visited the facility in March and May 2009.

- We talked with management and employees about their concerns.

- We toured the facility and observed employees at work.

- We spoke with employees confidentially about their health and asked if they had ever been diagnosed with MRSA.

- We discussed safety and health training at the facility and personal protective equipment use.

- We reviewed medical records of employees who reported current or past MRSA infections.

- We provided management and employees copies of the NIOSH Safety and Health Topic webpage *MRSA and the Workplace*.

- We reviewed the results of chemical and microbiological tests for metalworking fluids (MWFs) that were conducted from April 2005 to March 2009 by a third party.

- We collected bulk MWF from machine reservoirs and swab samples from machine and bathroom surfaces and tested them for the presence of MRSA.

## What NIOSH Found

- Three employees reported MRSA skin infections that were confirmed through laboratory testing conducted by their healthcare provider. We determined these infections were unlikely to be related to the workplace.

- The third party chemical and microbiological testing results from several MWF samples indicated that total bacteria levels are highly variable and poorly controlled.

- MRSA was not found in the bulk MWF or surface samples taken at the facility by NIOSH investigators.

- Many machines were not fitted with engineering controls or enclosures to keep MWF from splashing or misting.

## What Managers Can Do

- Ensure custodial staff keeps restrooms and hand-washing facilities clean.

- Encourage employees to report injuries to their supervisor in a timely manner.

- Urge employees to keep cuts or wounds covered with dry bandages to prevent the spread of MRSA infections while at work or home.

- Establish a comprehensive MWF maintenance program with designated supervision.

- Evaluate employee exposures to MWFs and evaluate the need for engineering controls and enclosures to machines to reduce exposure.

- Train employees on MWF health hazards, use of personal protective equipment, proper hygiene, and how to report health concerns.

- Include all employees exposed to MWF in a medical monitoring program.

## What Employees Can Do

- Tell management about any workplace injuries or health concerns that you think may be related to the workplace.

- Seek prompt medical care for any skin infections.

- Follow wound care instructions provided in the NIOSH guidance *MRSA and the Workplace* and as provided by your healthcare provider.

- Participate in training when provided.

- Use appropriate personal protective equipment such as gloves, sleeves, and aprons to reduce skin contact with MWFs.

- Wash MWFs off skin as soon as possible.

- Maintain good skin health through proper hygiene and use of moisturizers.

- Use a high efficiency particulate air (HEPA) filtered vacuum to remove dust, and use rags or cloths to wipe up excess MWF from parts and machines instead of using compressed air.

# SUMMARY

**It is unlikely that the three cases of MRSA among workers at the facility were related to workplace exposures. Although we did not isolate MRSA from the MWF in this facility, this route of exposure is plausible and warrants additional evaluation. We recommend that management assess the need for engineering controls to reduce exposure to MWF, and institute a comprehensive MWF maintenance program to reduce the potential for microbiological contamination.**

In February 2009, NIOSH received an HHE request from management at Positrol Inc. in Cincinnati, Ohio. The company was concerned because several workers had previously reported MRSA skin infections, and management wanted to determine if these infections were related to workplace exposures.

In March 2009, we visited Positrol and observed work processes. During the visit we held an opening conference, interviewed employees, and reviewed records. In May 2009, we collected bulk MWF samples and swab samples from machines and bathroom surfaces to test for the presence of MRSA bacteria.

Our investigation determined that three employees had previously been diagnosed with MRSA; however, these infections did not appear to be related to each other or to workplace exposures. The analysis of the bulk MWF and surface samples did not show the presence of MRSA. Our analysis of microbiological and pH tests conducted by a third party from April 2005 to March 2009 found that total bacterial levels in the MWF were highly variable and poorly controlled.

Many of the machines at the facility were not fitted with engineering controls or enclosures to prevent splashing or misting of MWF. We recommend that management evaluate employee exposures to MWF and, based on guidance outlined in this report, evaluate the need for engineering controls and enclosures to reduce exposure. We also recommend implementing a comprehensive MWF maintenance program to control bacteria, and encouraging employees to use appropriate PPE and practice good hygiene and wound management.

**Keywords:** NAICS 33515 (Cutting Tool and Machine Tool Accessory Manufacturing), metalworking fluid, methicillin-resistant *Staphylococcus aureus*, machine shop, MRSA

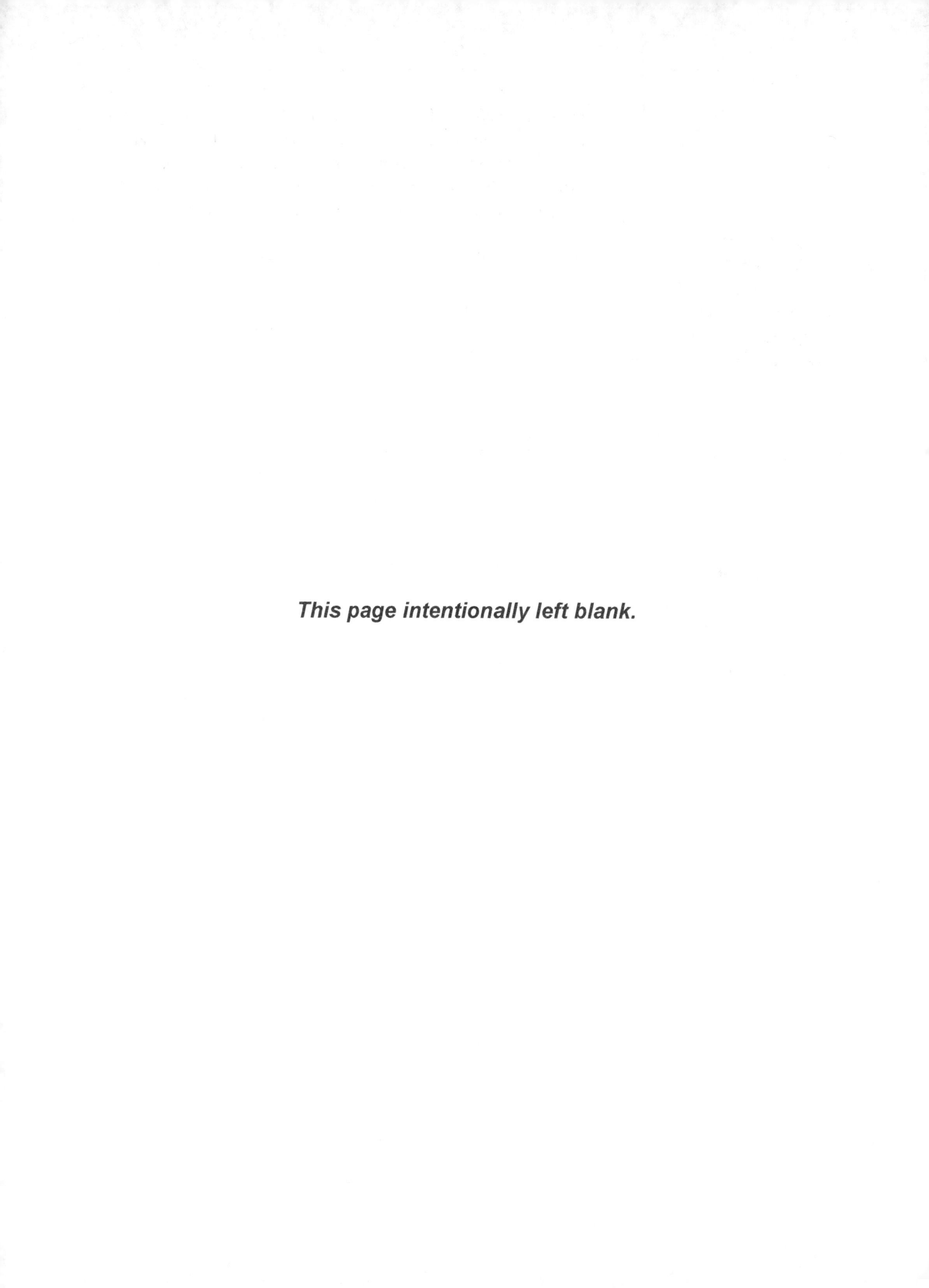

*This page intentionally left blank.*

# INTRODUCTION

In February 2009, NIOSH received a management request for an HHE at Positrol Inc. in Cincinnati, Ohio. The company submitted the HHE request because several employees had reported probable MRSA skin infections, and management wanted to determine if these infections were related to workplace exposures.

## Background

Positrol Inc. machines and produces a wide variety of workholding devices for industrial applications. Initial discussions with management upon receipt of the HHE request did not identify typical environmental risk factors for MRSA transmission such as shared shower facilities, towels, or locker rooms. We sent management the NIOSH document *MRSA and the Workplace* to provide background on MRSA infection and prevention strategies.

The facility, a one-story building, consists of office space and a shop floor. The various types of machining tools in the shop area include computer-numeric controlled, drilling, grinding, and lathing machines. Most machines use commercially available synthetic MWFs. Each machine has its own MWF reservoir. Biocides are not added to the MWFs to control the growth of microorganisms. The frequency of MWF addition or replacement varies at the discretion of the machine operator.

# ASSESSMENT

In response to the HHE request, we visited the facility on March 12 and May 14, 2009. On March 12, 2009, we held an opening meeting with management and employee representatives, followed by a tour of the facility. We talked with employees who agreed to confidential interviews, observed work procedures, and obtained medical records for three employees who self-reported current or prior infection with MRSA to confirm their diagnosis.

Management provided bacteria and pH testing results of MWFs conducted by a third party, dating from April 2005 to March 2009. To determine the amount of bacteria in the MWF, the third party company submerged a Sani Check® BF paddle (Biosan Laboratories, Inc., Warren, Michigan) in a sample of MWF. The paddle was incubated at 25°C–30°C for 24–36 hours. Bacterial growth on the paddle was then compared to a picture conversion chart to estimate the bacterial load in the MWF. From these results, it appeared that testing was conducted every 2–5 months on the machines.

On May 14, 2009, we returned to the facility and collected bulk MWF and swab surface samples in various locations for analysis of MRSA. We wore nitrile gloves while collecting samples and changed them out between samples to minimize the risk of cross-contamination. Bulk MWF samples were collected at the fluid nozzle of five machines by directing approximately 40 mL of MWF into a sterile polypropylene conical tube (Becton, Dickinson and Company, Franklin Lakes, New Jersey). Eleven swab samples were collected from the surfaces of five machines, men's shop bathroom, office area bathroom, lunchroom, and office area. Dry sterile foam-tipped applicator swabs (Puritan Medical Products Company, Guilford, Maine) were used to collect these samples. Samples were collected in a 100 cm² area using disposable 10 cm x 10 cm templates. After collection, swabs were placed in sterile polypropylene conical tubes. Table 1 provides a description of the samples collected.

**Table 1. Bulk and swab samples collected on May 14, 2009**

| Sample Type | Sample Location | Machine Serial Number | Comments |
|---|---|---|---|
| Bulk | Milwaukee K&T horizontal mill | 533-59 | Coolant rarely changed |
| Bulk | ROM 1 M20 milling machine | 533-92 | Coolant changed approximately 3 weeks before sampling |
| Bulk | OD grinder | 533-86 | Coolant rarely changed |
| Bulk | OD grinder | 533-50 | Coolant rarely changed |
| Bulk | LV 15 lathe | 533-78 | Coolant changed approximately 4 weeks before sampling |
| Swab | AVS lathe - flat surface above handle | 533-04 | Coolant rarely changed |
| Swab | Automatic grinder - flat surface next to handle | 533-15 | Coolant changed 3–5 days before sampling |
| Swab | Lathe - flat surface near handles | 533-88 | Coolant change unknown |
| Swab | Men's shop bathroom - large communal sink | — | — |
| Swab | Men's shop bathroom - next to stall one door handle | — | — |
| Swab | Women's bathroom adjacent to breakroom - sink | — | — |
| Swab | Breakroom - counter in front of microwave | — | — |
| Swab | Office area - desktop surface | — | — |
| Swab | ROM 1 M20 milling machine - surface next to handle on top cover | — | — |
| Swab | LV 15 Lathe - flat surface next to handle | — | — |
| Swab | Field blank | — | — |

All samples (bulk and swab) were placed in a cooler with ice and shipped overnight to Microbiology Specialists, Inc.® in Houston, Texas. The samples were swabbed onto BBL™ CHROMagar™ MRSA (BD-Diagnostic Systems, Sparks, Maryland), a selective and differential medium for the detection of MRSA. The media were held at 35°C in ambient conditions for 48 hours, but were read at 24-hour intervals. MRSA is identified on these media by the growth of mauve-colored colonies.

# RESULTS

## Industrial Hygiene

The microbiological test results we reviewed indicated that bacterial CFUs ranged from $<10^2$ to $10^7$ CFU/mL from 2005 to 2009. The pH of the MWFs ranged from 7.8 to 9.5. No obvious pattern was observed in these results over time.

No mauve-colored colonies were noted on the BBL CHROMagar media at 24 or 48 hours, indicating that MRSA was not isolated from any of the bulk and swab samples we collected.

## Interviews and Records Review

Of the 15 employees who worked on the machine shop floor, five participated in confidential interviews. Three employees reported being told by their physician that they had been infected with MRSA; two of these employees reported multiple infections and infections among family members over months to years. A review of their medical records determined that all three had been diagnosed with MRSA in the past by culture and sensitivity testing conducted at a clinical laboratory. Other issues raised included recurring sinus infections, lack of timely injury reporting, and concerns about using compressed air to clean off machines and parts, which generates dust and aerosols.

# DISCUSSION

MRSA refers to types of *Staphylococcus aureus (S. aureus)* bacteria that are resistant to several antibiotics, including methicillin. Approximately 25%–35% of the U.S. population is colonized (a person who carries a bacteria on his or her body but does not exhibit signs of disease) by *S. aureus*, while an estimated 1.5% is colonized by MRSA [Gorwitz et al. 2008]. Community-acquired MRSA infections usually occur as skin and/or soft tissue infections in otherwise healthy people. Historically, outbreaks have been reported in schools, correctional facilities, and military barracks [Lindenmayer et al. 1998; CDC 2003a,b; Zinderman et al. 2004; Cohen 2005]. Factors that have been associated with the spread of MRSA skin infections include close skin-to-skin contact, contamination of skin whose integrity has been compromised through cuts or abrasions, contact with contaminated items and surfaces such as soiled bandages or towels, crowded living conditions, and poor hygiene.

MRSA was not detected in any of the swab or bulk samples that we collected. As part of our investigation, we collected bulk and swab samples on machines where MRSA-infected employees worked as well as on machines where employees did not report MRSA infections. In a review of the scientific literature, we identified no publications that linked exposure to MWFs with MRSA infections; however, it is plausible that this type of bacteria could grow in a water-based synthetic MWF environment [Weissfeld 2009].

Our review of prior test results for bacteria in Positrol MWFs found that concentrations of bacteria were very high at times (up to $10^7$ CFU/mL). Although NIOSH has no RELs for bacteria and fungi in MWFs, the HSE in the United Kingdom has provided guidance on this issue. The HSE recommends keeping bacteria levels in MWF below $10^3$ CFU/mL. If bacteria levels are between $10^3$ and $10^6$ CFU/mL in the MWF, the HSE recommends cleaning the system or changing the biocide regimen. If bacteria levels are greater than $10^6$ CFU/mL, they recommend that the employer immediately drain the MWFs and clean the machine [HSE 2006]. Additional guidance from the HSE on MWFs can be found at http://www.hse.gov.uk/metalworking/ecoshh.htm. The HSE recommends testing bacteria at least once a week [HSE 2006].

Although we did not monitor the air for MWFs during our evaluation, we observed some conditions that may lead to employee airborne MWF exposures. Specifically, many tooling machines that use MWFs were neither enclosed nor fitted with

# DISCUSSION
(CONTINUED)

engineering controls that would help reduce concentrations of MWF mists. Additionally, we observed that many employees did not wear gloves when working with MWFs.

Substantial scientific evidence indicates that employees currently exposed to MWF aerosols have an increased risk of respiratory (lung) and skin diseases. These health effects vary based on the type of MWF, route of exposure, concentration, and length of exposure [NIOSH 1998b]. The NIOSH REL for MWF aerosols is 0.5 mg/m$^3$ for total MWF particulates and 0.4 mg/m$^3$ for the thoracic particulate mass, as a TWA concentration for up to 10 hours per day during a 40-hour workweek. The NIOSH REL is intended to prevent or greatly reduce respiratory disorders associated with MWF exposure. Some employees have developed work-related asthma, HP, or other adverse respiratory effects when exposed to MWFs at concentrations below the NIOSH REL [NIOSH 1998a,b]. In addition, limiting dermal (skin) exposure is critical to preventing allergic and irritant disorders related to MWF exposure. In most metalworking operations, it is technologically feasible to limit MWF aerosol exposures to 0.4 mg/m$^3$ or less by using engineering controls. NIOSH also recommends medical monitoring for employees exposed to MWF. Medical monitoring is needed for the early identification of employees who develop symptoms of MWF-related conditions such as HP, asthma, and dermatitis [NIOSH 1998a,b]. If all employees cannot be included in a medical monitoring program, priority should be given to those at high risk; for example, those exposed to MWF aerosol concentrations above a designated level such as half the REL [NIOSH 1998a,b]. Medical monitoring consists of preplacement and periodic examinations under the medical direction and supervision of a qualified physician or other qualified health care provider as determined by appropriate state regulations. These examinations should be provided to employees at no cost.

More detailed information on administering a medical monitoring program for MWF exposure is provided in Appendix A as well as information on health effects associated with MWFs, microbiological contaminants, and occupational exposure limits. Appendix B is a copy of the State of Washington Department of Labor and Industries Technical Report 55-7-2001, "Prevention of Skin Problems when Working with Metal Working Fluids." This document provides some information on how MWFs may cause dermatitis and how to prevent it. The NIOSH criteria document for MWFs provides information about respiratory and dermal

# DISCUSSION
## (CONTINUED)

health effects of MWFs [NIOSH 1998a]. Links to both of these documents and other useful websites that provide guidelines for controlling employee exposures to MWFs and MWF maintenance are available on the NIOSH Metalworking Fluids topic page at http://www.cdc.gov/niosh/topics/metalworking.

# CONCLUSIONS

Based on the absence of risk factors commonly associated with occupational outbreaks of MRSA infection (contact with contaminated bandages or towels, crowding living conditions, shared shower facilities, and poor hygiene), negative MRSA results in MWF bulk samples and environmental swab sampling, and evidence of household transmission among two of three infected employees, we conclude that the cases of MRSA reported at the facility were likely not related to occupational exposure. However, NIOSH investigators identified many machines used at the facility that are not enclosed or fitted with local exhaust ventilation to control employee exposures to MWFs. Additionally, our review of past environmental sampling results revealed inadequate control of biological growth in the MWFs at the facility.

# RECOMMENDATIONS

Based on our findings, we recommend the actions listed below to create a more healthful workplace. We encourage Positrol Inc. to use these recommendations to develop an action plan based, if possible, on the hierarchy of controls approach. This approach groups actions by their likely effectiveness in reducing or removing hazards. In most cases, the preferred approach is to eliminate hazardous materials or processes and install engineering controls to reduce exposure or shield employees. Until such controls are in place, or if they are not effective or feasible, administrative measures and/or personal protective equipment may be needed.

## Administrative Controls

Administrative controls are management-dictated work practices and policies to reduce or prevent exposures to workplace hazards. The effectiveness of administrative changes in work practices for controlling workplace hazards is dependent on management commitment and employee acceptance. Regular monitoring and reinforcement are necessary to ensure that control policies and procedures are not circumvented in the name of convenience or production.

# Recommendations
## (CONTINUED)

1. Because MRSA transmission in the community will continue to occur, the following recommendations are offered to help prevent further MRSA skin infections. Additional information about MRSA in the workplace can be found at http://www.cdc.gov/niosh/topics/mrsa/.

   a. Employees should report injuries and infections that are potentially related to work to their supervisor.

   b. Employees should keep draining wounds covered with clean, dry bandages. If wounds are covered, isolation of infected employees is not necessary.

   c. Employees should wash their hands regularly with soap and water or alcohol-based hand gel. This is the single-most important measure to help prevent a wide variety of infections.

   d. Employees should maintain good personal hygiene with regular bathing.

   e. Employees should not share items that may become contaminated with wound drainage, such as towels, clothing, or razors.

   f. The company should clean equipment, surfaces, and restroom and hand-washing facilities with detergent-based cleaners or EPA-registered disinfectants that are labeled as effective in removing bacteria from the environment. It is important to read label directions thoroughly and ensure all products are used safely and appropriately. A list of EPA-registered products effective against MRSA is located at http://www.epa.gov/oppad001/list_h_mrsa_vre.pdf.

2. Develop a comprehensive MWF program. NIOSH and OSHA provide examples of comprehensive MWF programs [NIOSH 1998a; OSHA 1999]. Both of these programs outline aspects of MWF management including safety and health training, employee participation, environmental monitoring, hazard prevention and control, and medical monitoring.

   a. Include all employees exposed to MWF in a medical monitoring program [NIOSH 1998a,b]. This is necessary because maintaining MWF concentrations below the NIOSH REL does not remove all risk for skin or respiratory disease among exposed employees.

# RECOMMENDATIONS
(CONTINUED)

Primary prevention efforts to control inhalation and skin exposure to MWFs should be done in addition to the medical monitoring program. NIOSH publication 98-116, *What You Need to Know about Occupational Exposure to MWFs* at http://www.cdc.gov/niosh/pdfs/98-116.pdf provides guidelines for administering a medical monitoring program [NIOSH 1998b].

b. Train employees in the health hazards associated with MWFs, use of PPE, proper hygiene, and procedures for reporting adverse health effects. Additional information on these topics can be found in the NIOSH publications on MWFs [NIOSH 1998a,b].

c. Follow your MWF supplier's and the HSE's recommendations for MWF maintenance [HSE 2006].

- Keep microbial growth under control by adding the proper amount of biocides before problems develop.

- Keep MWF pH at 8.8–9.2 or as recommended by your supplier.

- Maintain bacterial concentrations below $10^3$ CFU/mL and fungal levels at <100 CFU/mL [HSE 2006].

d. To lessen respiratory exposure, do not use compressed air to clean dust and excess MWF off machines or parts. Alternatives include the use of a HEPA filtered vacuum for dust and rags or cloths to wipe up excess MWF.

# REFERENCES

CDC (Centers for Disease Control and Prevention) [2003a]. Methicillin-resistant *Staphylococcus aureus* infections in correctional facilities–Georgia, California, and Texas, 2001–2003. MMWR *52*(41):992–996.

CDC (Centers for Disease Control and Prevention) [2003b]. Outbreaks of community-associated methicillin-resistant *Staphylococcus aureus* skin infections–Los Angeles County, California, 2002–2003. MMWR *52*(5):88.

Cohen PR [2005]. Cutaneous community-acquired methicillin-resistant *Staphylococcus aureus* infection in participants of athletic activities. South Med J 98(6):596–602.

# REFERENCES
(CONTINUED)

Gorwitz RJ, Kruszon-Moran D, McAllister SK, McQuillan G, McDougal LK, Fosheim GE, Jensen BJ, Killgore G, Tenover FC, Kuehnert MJ [2008]. Changes in the prevalence of nasal colonization with *Staphylococcus aureus* in the United States, 2001–2004. J Infect Dis *197*(9):1226–1234.

HSE [2006]. Managing sumps and bacterial contamination–control approach 4. COSHH essentials for machining with metalworking fluids. [http://www.hse.gov.uk/pubns/guidance/mw05.pdf]. Date accessed: December 2009.

Lindenmayer JM, Schoenfeld S, O'Grady R, Carney JK 1998]. Methicillin-resistant *Staphylococcus aureus* in a high school wrestling team and the surrounding community. Arch Intern Med *58*(8):895–899.

NIOSH [1998a]. Criteria for a recommended standard: occupational exposure to metalworking fluids. Cincinnati, OH: U.S. Department of Health and Human Services, Centers for Disease Control and Prevention, National Institute for Occupational Safety and Health, DHHS (NIOSH) Publication No. 98-102.

NIOSH [1998b]. What you need to know about occupational exposure to metalworking fluids. Cincinnati, OH: U.S. Department of Health and Human Services, Centers for Disease Control and Prevention, National Institute for Occupational Safety and Health, DHHS (NIOSH) Publication No. 98-116.

OSHA [1999]. Metalworking Fluids: Safety and Health Best Practices Manual. [http://www.osha.gov/SLTC/metalworkingfluids/metalworkingfluids_manual.html]. Date accessed: January 2010.

Weissfeld A [2009]. Telephone conversation on April 29, 2009, between A. Weissfeld, Microbiology Specialists Inc., and T. Niemeier, Division of Surveillance, Hazard Evaluations and Field Studies, National Institute for Occupational Safety and Health, Centers for Disease Control and Prevention, U.S. Department of Health and Human Services.

Zinderman CE, Conner B, Malakooti MA [2004]. Community-acquired methicillin-resistant *Staphylococcus aureus* among military recruits. Emerg Infect Dis *10*(5):941–944.

Metalworking fluids are complex mixtures used to cool, lubricate, and remove metal chips from tools and metal parts during machining of metal stock. Machining processes may include grinding, cutting, or boring operations. The four types of MWFs include straight oils, soluble oils, semisynthetics, and synthetics [NIOSH 1998a,b; OSHA 1999]. Most straight oils are highly refined products of petroleum stocks or animal, marine, and vegetable oils. Straight oils do not contain nor are they diluted with water. Other types of MWFs are water-based mixtures that may require dilution. Both soluble oils (oil-based, with emulsifiers) and semisynthetic fluids (oil emulsion, with large amounts of water) contain some oil, while synthetic fluids are totally water-based products. MWFs often contain a mixture of other substances including biocides, corrosion inhibitors, metal fines, tramp oils, and biological contaminants [NIOSH 1998a]. Selection of a specific MWF is based on the requirements of the task. For example, straight oils are cutting oils and prevent rusting of the metal, while water soluble oils cool and lubricate the metal parts [OSHA 1999].

The term MWF aerosol refers to the mist generated during machining, which may contain a variety of substances including any component of the MWF, additives to the MWF, contaminants of the MWF such as tramp oils or metals, and biological contaminants such as bacteria and fungi, as well as their byproducts such as endotoxin, exotoxins, and mycotoxins. Exposure to MWFs can result from inhaling aerosols or from skin contact due to touching contaminated surfaces, handling parts and equipment, splashing of fluids, and settling of MWF aerosol on the skin [NIOSH 1998a,b]. Inhalation of MWF aerosols may irritate the throat (e.g., sore, burning throat), nose (e.g., runny nose, congestion, and nosebleeds), and lungs (e.g., cough, wheezing, increased phlegm production, and shortness of breath). MWF aerosol exposure has been associated with chronic bronchitis, asthma, HP, and worsening of pre-existing respiratory problems. HP is a spectrum of granulomatous, interstitial lung diseases that occurs after repeated inhalation and sensitization to a wide variety of microbial agents (i.e., bacteria, fungi, amoebae), animal proteins, and low-molecular weight chemical antigens [CDC 1996; Kreiss and Cox-Ganser 1997; Zacharisen et al. 1998]. Skin contact with MWFs may cause allergic contact dermatitis and/or irritant contact dermatitis depending on the chemical composition of the fluid, types of additives and contaminants contained in the MWFs, type of metal being machined (e.g., nickel or chromium), and the exposed individual's tendency for developing allergies. Petroleum-based products may cause occupational acne [WISHA 2001]. Certain chemical additives, such as those with a low or high pH, irritate the skin upon direct contact. Strong detergents and hand cleansers may also cause dermatitis or aggravate an existing condition.

## Mineral Oils

Mineral oils are major components of many MWFs and can contain a complex mixture of aromatic, naphthenic, and straight- or branched-chain paraffinic hydrocarbons, as well as various additives and impurities. In addition to the general exposure criteria for MWFs cited above, there are criteria specifically for the mineral oil components of MWFs. Occupational exposure to mineral oil concentrations in air (often called mineral oil mists) is limited by the OSHA PEL and NIOSH REL to 5 mg/m$^3$; NIOSH also recommends a STEL of 10 mg/m$^3$ [29 CFR 1910.1000; NIOSH 2005].

Inhalation of mineral oil mist in high concentrations may cause pulmonary effects (e.g , lipoid pneumonitis), although few cases have been reported [Proudfit and Van Orstrand 1950]. Prolonged exposure to mineral oil mist may also cause dermatitis. Persons with pre-existing skin disorders may be more susceptible to these effects. Early epidemiological studies linked cancers of the skin and scrotum with exposure to mineral oils [IARC 1982]. It is thought that the presence of PAHs and/or additives with carcinogenic properties was responsible for cancer causation in the older MWFs. Modern mineral oils are highly refined, which has reduced the concentrations of PAHs found in older, poorly refined mineral oils. For uncharacterized mineral oils containing additives and impurities, the IARC determined that there is sufficient evidence for carcinogenicity to humans, based on epidemiologic studies; however, IARC has determined that for highly refined mineral oils, there is inadequate evidence for carcinogenicity to humans [IARC 1987].

## Microbial Contaminants

Synthetic, semisynthetic, and soluble oil MWFs are diluted with water. Hence, they can provide a breeding ground for bacteria if an inadequate amount of biocide is added. High temperature and low pH and the presence of metals can favor bacterial growth. Levels of microbial contamination indicate the cleanliness or degree of maintenance of the MWF. However, adding too much biocide may result in biocide-resistant strains of bacteria. Inhaling MWF aerosols containing bacteria may result in respiratory problems. Employees with broken skin may develop skin infections if they have contact with MWF contaminated with bacteria. The outer cell walls of Gram-negative bacteria in MWFs may release lipopolysaccharide compounds called endotoxin when the bacteria die or multiply [Olenchock 1997]. Endotoxin are believed to cause adverse respiratory effects such as chronic bronchitis and asthma. Adding biocides to water contaminated with bacteria may result in the release of endotoxin by dead organisms.

Insufficient data exist to determine what constitutes a safe level of microbial contamination in MWF – either in terms of species present, absolute number of colony forming units, or microbial components. Rylander and Jacobs have suggested an occupational threshold concentration equivalent to 100 endotoxin units/m$^3$ of air to prevent airway inflammation [Rylander and Jacobs 1997]. However, the concentration of endotoxin in bulk samples of MWF cannot be extrapolated to an airborne concentration because the airborne concentration depends on how much of the MWF is aerosolized. Contaminated water in MWF may also contain fungi. Fungi may infect susceptible hosts such as immunocompromised persons. Cephalosporium, a genus commonly isolated from MWFs, has reportedly caused HP. Fungi may also produce toxic metabolites called mycotoxins. When contaminated MWF is replaced, some of the bacteria may remain and proliferate within a short period if the system is not adequately cleaned. At this time there is insufficient health data to recommend a specific limit for bacterial or fungal contamination in MWF.

Some researchers have suggested that well-maintained MWFs should have bacterial concentrations below 10$^6$ CFU/mL of fluid [Rossmore and Rossmore 1994]. In a study of 19 small machine shops, Korean and Canadian occupational health professionals found that a pH >8.5 (a pH of 9.0–9.5 was found to be preferable for controlling the growth of microorganisms) and avoiding contamination of the MWFs with tramp oils and foreign substances would help maintain lower endotoxin levels in MWF sumps [Park et al. 2001]. The HSE in the United Kingdom has also provided guidance on control of bacteria in MWFs. The HSE recommends keeping bacteria levels in MWF below $10^3$ CFU/mL. If bacteria levels are between $10^3$ and $10^6$ CFU/mL in the MWF, the HSE recommends cleaning the system or changing the biocide. If bacteria levels are greater than $10^6$ CFU/mL, they recommend that the employer immediately drain the MWFs and clean the machine [HSE 2006]. Additional guidance from HSE on MWFs can be found at http://www.hse.gov.uk/metalworking/ecoshh.htm. The HSE recommends testing bacteria once a week [HSE 2006].

## Occupational Exposure Limits

NIOSH recommends limiting exposures to MWF aerosols to 0.4 mg/m$^3$ for the thoracic particulate mass, as a TWA concentration for up to 10 hours per day during a 40-hour workweek [NIOSH 1998a]. The NIOSH REL is intended to prevent or greatly reduce respiratory disorders associated with MWF exposure. Some employees have developed work-related asthma, HP, or other adverse respiratory effects when exposed to MWFs at concentrations below the NIOSH REL. Limiting exposure to MWF aerosols is also prudent because certain MWF exposures have been associated with various cancers. In addition, limiting dermal (skin) exposure is critical to preventing allergic and irritant disorders related to MWF exposure. In most metalworking operations, it is technologically feasible to limit MWF aerosol exposures to 0.4 mg/m$^3$ or less. NIOSH also recommends medical monitoring for employees exposed to MWF. Medical monitoring is needed for the early identification of employees who develop symptoms of MWF-related conditions such as HP, asthma, and dermatitis. NIOSH recommends that all employees exposed to MWFs at over half the REL receive medical monitoring.

## Medical Monitoring

Medical monitoring is secondary prevention. Primary preventive measures such as engineering controls are the most effective and important methods of preventing illness. However, medical monitoring does have a place in identifying employees who develop symptoms of MWF-related conditions such as asthma or dermatitis. All employees exposed to MWF above half of the NIOSH REL should be included in the medical monitoring, and all employees with exposure may benefit from medical monitoring.

Supervision of the program should be done by a physician or other health professional who is knowledgeable about the respiratory protection program and the identification and management of MWF-related respiratory conditions and skin diseases. The employer should provide the health professional current and previous job descriptions, hazardous exposures and their measurements, the type of PPE used, relevant material safety data sheets, and applicable safety and health standards.

Medical monitoring should be provided at no cost to the employees, and the physician's recommended restrictions and accommodations should be adhered to. A monitoring program should include the following components:

1. Initial or preplacement exams that consist of a standardized symptom questionnaire, medical history, and skin exam, at a minimum. Spirometry would be useful to establish baseline lung function for future comparison.

2. Periodic exams that include a brief standardized symptom questionnaire. Skin exam and spirometry may also be useful. The frequency of exams should be based on the frequency and severity of health effects. Employees who do experience health effects possibly related to MWF exposure should be given more detailed exams.

3. A written report from the physician that includes the results of any tests performed, the physician's opinion about any medical condition that may increase the risk of disease from exposures in the workplace, any recommended restrictions or accommodations, and recommendations for further evaluation or treatment. The physician should provide the employer with a written report that includes any recommended restrictions and a statement that the employee was informed of the results of the exam and of any medical condition that requires further evaluation or treatment. No information regarding specific findings or diagnoses should be released to the employer without a signed information release from the employee.

# References

CDC (Centers for Disease Control and Prevention) [1996]. Biopsy-confirmed hypersensitivity pneumonitis in automobile production workers exposed to metalworking fluids – Michigan. MMWR 45(28):606–610.

CFR. Code of Federal Regulations. Washington, DC: U.S. Government Printing Office, Office of the Federal Register.

HSE [2006]. Managing sumps and bacterial contamination – control approach 4. COSHH essentials for machining with metalworking fluids. [http://www.hse.gov.uk/pubns/guidance/mw05.pdf]. Date accessed: December 2009.

IARC [1982]. Monographs on the evaluation of the carcinogenic risk of chemicals to humans: chemicals, industrial processes and industries associated with cancer in humans. Suppl. 4. Lyon, France: World Health Organization, International Agency for Research on Cancer, pp. 227–228.

IARC [1987]. Monographs on the evaluation of the carcinogenic risk of chemicals to humans, overall evaluations of carcinogenicity: an updating of IARC monographs vols. 1 to 42. Suppl. 7. Lyon, France: World Health Organization, International Agency for Research on Cancer, pp. 252–254.

Kreiss K, Cox-Ganser J [1997]. Metalworking fluid associated hypersensitivity pneumonitis: a workshop summary. Am J Ind Med 32(4):423–432.

NIOSH [1998a]. Criteria for a recommended standard: Occupational exposure to metalworking fluids. Cincinnati, OH: U.S. Department of Health and Human Services, Centers for Disease Control and Prevention, National Institute for Occupational Safety and Health, DHHS (NIOSH) Publication No. 98-102.

NIOSH [1998b]. What you need to know about occupational exposure to metalworking fluids. Cincinnati, OH: U.S. Department of Health and Human Services, Centers for Disease Control and Prevention, National Institute for Occupational Safety and Health, DHHS (NIOSH) Publication No. 98-116.

NIOSH [2005]. NIOSH pocket guide to chemical hazards. Barsan ME, ed. Cincinnati, OH: U.S. Department of Health and Human Services, Centers for Disease Control and Prevention, National Institute for Occupational Safety and Health, DHHS (NIOSH) Publication No. 2005-149.

Olenchock S [1997]. Airborne endotoxin. In: Hurst CJ, Knudsen GR, McInerney MJ, Stetzenbach LD, Walter MV, eds. Manual of Environmental Microbiology. Washington, DC: American Society for Microbiology Press, pp. 661–665.

OSHA [1999]. Metalworking fluids safety and health best practices manual. [http://www.osha.gov/SLTC/metalworkingfluids/metalworkingfluids_manual.html]. Date accessed: December 2009.

Park D, Teschke K, Bartlett K [2001]. A model for predicting endotoxin concentrations in metalworking fluid sumps in small machine shops. Ann Occup Hyg 45(7):569–576.

Proudfit JP, Van Ordstrand HS [1950]. Chronic lipid pneumonia following occupational exposure. AMA Arch Ind Hyg Occup Med 1(1):105–111.

Rossmoore LA, Rossmoore HW [1994]. Metalworking fluid microbiology. In: Metalworking Fluids. Byers J ed. New York, NY: Marcel Dekker, Inc. pp. 247–271.

Rylander R, Jacobs RR [1997]. Endotoxin in the environment. Intl J Occup Environ Health 3(1):S1-S31.

WISHA [2001]. Preventing occupational dermatitis. Olympia, WA: Washington State Department of Labor and Industries, Safety & Health Assessment & Research for Prevention (SHARP) Publication No. 56-01-1999.

Zacharisen MC, Kadambi AR, Schlueter DP, Kurup VP, Shack JB, Fox JL, Anderson HA, Fink JN [1998]. The spectrum of respiratory disease associated with exposure to metal working fluids. J Occup Environ Med 40(7):640–647.

# Appendix B: Prevention of Skin Problems when Working with Metal Working Fluids*

## Introduction

Metal working fluids are industrial coolants and lubricants used to reduce friction and heat generated with the machining, grinding and fabrication operations of metal products and to lubricate during metalworking operations. The fluids prolong the life of machines, carry away metal chips and protect the surfaces of the metal being processed.

There are three main types of MWFs:

- insoluble fluids (straight or neat oils),
- soluble oils (oil in water emulsions) and
- synthetic fluids.

These fluids can have additives that are corrosion inhibitors, emulsifiers, anti- foaming agents, preservatives and biocides. The formula of oil used depends on the raw material or cutting operation to be carried out. Straight or neat oils are not commonly found in machine shops as they once were.

## Skin Problems

MWFs can be irritating to the skin. Skin problems include mechanical trauma to the skin, infections, oil acne, folliculitis and irritant and allergic dermatitis.

### Mechanical Trauma

Small cuts to the skin from metal shavings (swarf) are a common injury. These cuts can become infected as a result from contact with MWFs fluids contaminated with microbial organisms.

### Folliculitis and Oil Acne

Exposure to straight oils can result in folliculitis (inflammation of the hair follicles) after having direct contact of oil with the skin. Exposed skin or skin under clothing heavily contaminated with oil results in blocked skin follicles. Blocked follicles can range in appearance from red irritation around hair follicles, small black plugged pores to large pustules. This problem can be found on the neck, hands, arms and thighs. If a employees has acne when starting a job working around MWFs, the fluids on the skin may make the acne worse.

---

\*      Safety and Health Assessment and Research for Prevention Technical Report: 55-7-2001. Washington State Department of Labor and Industries. 1-888-66-SHARP. [www.lni.wa.gov/sharp/derm].

## Irritant Dermatitis

This is the most common type of skin problem due to exposure to MWFs. Soluble and synthetic metal working fluids are strong alkaline solutions (pH of approximately 9 - very basic) containing numerous additives and solvents. These solutions remove protective oils in the skin and damage proteins in its outer layer. The result is damage to the natural skin barrier, which causes a decrease in the water content of the skin. This can cause dry, thickened, fissured and inflamed skin, especially on the palms of the hands. The hands and forearms can develop dry, scaly and inflamed patches. Infrequently, very small fluid-filled blisters can also develop on the hands and fingers. Small cuts in the skin from metal pieces allow more penetration n of irritant fluids and contribute to irritant dermatitis. The type and concentration of fluid used, duration of exposure during the work period, and the presence of pre-existing skin disease (eczema or severe dry skin) all contribute to the development of dermatitis.

## Allergic Dermatitis

This is less common than irritant dermatitis. The additives in MWFs such as biocides, preservatives, corrosion inhibitors, amines and the impurities from metal (chrome, nickel), act as allergens and can cause an allergic reaction in some susceptible individuals. When skin is irritated, these allergens can penetrate more easily through the damaged skin barrier. A person who has developed an allergy to additives or impurities can have lesions that resemble irritant dermatitis, usually on the fingers and hands, but the lesions do not clear when the person is away from the job (vacation) or with treatment. This person needs to be evaluated with patch testing to the components of MWFs (additives and metal impurities) to see if there is an allergen responsible for the persistent skin reaction.

## *Prevention of Dermatitis*

A primary method for the prevention of skin problems is to avoid contact with MWFs. Although it is impossible to avoid all contact with the fluids, the contact can be minimized and the irritancy of the fluids can be controlled.

## Environment

Here are some ways to decrease contact with the fluids:

- keep the work area clean, including the machines, from machining fluids and grime, and
- have functioning splashguards on the machines.

The irritancy of the fluids can be minimized by:

- changing to a less irritating MWF if feasible,
- correct dilution of the additives in the fluids,

- maintaining MWFs at the manufacturer-specified concentration and pH,

- ensuring the cleanliness of the fluids by recirculating and filtering/straining them to remove swarf and other solid contaminants, and

- avoiding the use of fluids that have become contaminated with excessive microbial organisms.

## Employees

Those working with MWFs can also help prevent developing dermatitis by:

- wearing clean clothes while on the job,

- laundering clothing that becomes contaminated with MWFs,

- avoiding placing MWF-soaked rags in pockets,

- wearing protective aprons, and

- wearing protective nitrile gloves (avoid latex because of the potential of developing an allergic reaction). Because of the nature of some jobs (fast rotating parts on a machine), wearing gloves may not be possible.

Personal cleanliness is necessary to remove irritating fluids before skin problems develop. This can be accomplished by the following measures:

- Washing hands with mild, nonabrasive soaps to remove fluids. Soiled skin areas should be washed at least twice during the workday.

- Never use cleaning solvents to wash the skin to remove fluids. These solvents increase the damage caused by irritating MWFs by removing even more protective oils in the skin.

- Wiping off hands during the day with towels that are not contaminated with fluids or swarf. Disposable paper towels should be considered.

Protecting the skin from the irritant effects of MWFs also requires keeping the skin in good shape.

- Use moisturizers before and after work. Products that are thick creams or ointments work best. These products may seem greasy but can heal the skin faster and offer more protection than thinner, water-based formulations. Working the moisturizer cream into the skin and wearing clean, thin cotton gloves for a couple of hours or wearing the gloves to bed can also speed the recovery of dry, fissured, irritated skin. Inexpensive 100% petroleum jelly works as a good moisturizing agent and has no added fragrance or preservatives. There are products on the market that are creamy petroleum jelly formulations and are easier to apply to the skin.

- Skin barrier creams have not shown to be as effective as claimed in preventing penetration of irritants and avoiding hand dermatitis. Silicone-based barrier creams are available but require vigilant use every few hours to help decrease contact of irritants with the skin.

- Using a mild soap at home can protect the skin from further damage.

## Treatment of Skin Problems from Metal Working Fluids

Prevention is the key to avoiding skin problems. However, despite all efforts, skin problems from MWFs may develop. The longer the skin problem has been present, the harder it is treat and to clear. Therefore, it is important to seek medical evaluation early if problems develop. The following skin problems may require the evaluation by a dermatologist or occupational medicine physician:

- severe oil acne or folliculitis,

- skin infections,

- severe irritated or fissured skin,

- persistent eczema or blisters, which may be irritant or allergic dermatitis. Occasionally, a person may require patch testing to determine if there is an allergic component to the skin problem. This usually is required when the skin problem does not respond to treatment.

# Acknowledgments and Availability of Report

The Hazard Evaluations and Technical Assistance Branch (HETAB) of the National Institute for Occupational Safety and Health (NIOSH) conducts field investigations of possible health hazards in the workplace. These investigations are conducted under the authority of Section 20(a)(6) of the Occupational Safety and Health Act of 1970, 29 U.S.C. 669(a)(6) which authorizes the Secretary of Health and Human Services, following a written request from any employer or authorized representative of employees, to determine whether any substance normally found in the place of employment has potentially toxic effects in such concentrations as used or found. HETAB also provides, upon request, technical and consultative assistance to federal, state, and local agencies; labor; industry; and other groups or individuals to control occupational health hazards and to prevent related trauma and disease.

The findings and conclusions in this report are those of the authors and do not necessarily represent the views of NIOSH. Mention of any company or product does not constitute endorsement by NIOSH. In addition, citations to websites external to NIOSH do not constitute NIOSH endorsement of the sponsoring organizations or their programs or products. Furthermore, NIOSH is not responsible for the content of these websites. All Web addresses referenced in this document were accessible as of the publication date.

This report was prepared by John Gibbins and Todd Niemeier of HETAB, Division of Surveillance, Hazard Evaluations and Field Studies. Medical field assistance was provided by Marie de Perio. Health communication assistance was provided by Stefanie Evans. Editorial assistance was provided by Ellen Galloway. Desktop publishing was performed by Robin Smith.

Copies of this report have been sent to employee and management representatives at Positrol Inc., the state health department, and the Occupational Safety and Health Administration Regional Office. This report is not copyrighted and may be freely reproduced. The report may be viewed and printed at http://www.cdc.gov/niosh/hhe/. Copies may be purchased from the National Technical Information Service at 5825 Port Royal Road, Springfield, Virginia 22161.

**Below is a recommended citation for this report:**
NIOSH [2009]. Health hazard evaluation report: evaluation of Methicillin-resistant *Staphylococcus aureus* (MRSA) cases among employees at a workholding manufacturing facility, Cincinnati, OH. By Gibbins J, Niemeier T. Cincinnati, OH: U.S. Department of Health and Human Services, Centers for Disease Control and Prevention, National Institute for Occupational Safety and Health, NIOSH HETA No. 2009-0098-3103

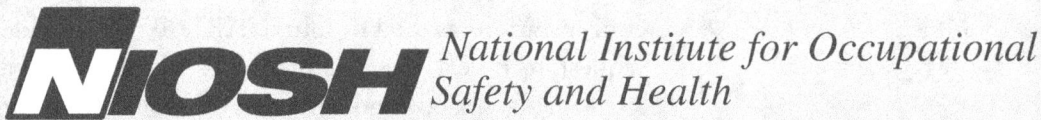

*National Institute for Occupational Safety and Health*

# Delivering on the Nation's promise: Safety and health at work for all people through research and prevention.

To receive NIOSH documents or information about occupational safety and health topics, contact NIOSH at:

**1-800-CDC-INFO** (1-800-232-4636)

TTY: 1-888-232-6348

E-mail: cdcinfo@cdc.gov

or visit the NIOSH web site at: **www.cdc.gov/niosh.**

For a monthly update on news at NIOSH, subscribe to NIOSH eNews by visiting **www.cdc.gov/niosh/eNews.**

SAFER • HEALTHIER • PEOPLE™

www.ingramcontent.com/pod-product-compliance
Lightning Source LLC
Chambersburg PA
CBHW080941290526
45795CB00007BA/2855